DIABETES BREAKFAST RECIPES COOKBOOK 2024

THE ULTIMATE GUIDE TO REVERSE DIABETES

PAM J. RIOS

embodied in critical reviews and certain other noncommercial uses permitted by copyright law.

This book is intended as a guide to adopting the Mediterranean diet for diabetes. While every effort has been made to ensure the accuracy of the information provided, the author and publisher shall not be held responsible for any omissions, errors, or damages arising from the use of this book.

The recipes, nutritional information, and dietary recommendations in this book are intended for informational purposes only and should not substitute professional medical advice or treatment. It is recommended that readers consult their healthcare providers before making any significant changes to their diet or lifestyle.

Any unauthorised use, distribution, or reproduction of this book without the expressed written consent of the copyright holder is strictly prohibited.

TABLE OF CONTENTS

INTRODUCTION

Welcome to the Diabetes Breakfast Recipes Cookbook 2024, a comprehensive guide to delicious and nutritious breakfast options for individuals with diabetes. In this book, you will find a collection of carefully crafted recipes that are designed to help you manage your blood sugar levels while enjoying a satisfying and wholesome breakfast. Whether you're looking for quick and easy options for busy mornings or indulgent weekend treats, this cookbook has got you covered. With detailed nutritional information and practical tips for meal planning, this book is a valuable resource for anyone looking to start their day off right while managing their diabetes. Let's start cooking and savoring the most important meal of the day!

During my research and studying of diabetes, I met a young woman named Sarah who was diagnosed with diabetes at the age of 25. Despite the initial shock and fear, she was determined to take control of her health and manage her condition the best way she could. One of the biggest challenges she faced was figuring out what to eat for breakfast that would help stabilize her blood sugar levels and keep her satisfied throughout the morning. That was how she contacted me.

After countless hours of research and experimentation in the kitchen, Sarah and I discovered a variety of delicious and nutritious breakfast recipes that not only kept her blood sugar in check, but also left her feeling energized and ready to take on the day. From smoothie bowls and oatmeal to egg dishes and homemade granola, we found that there were plenty of options for a diabetes-friendly breakfast that didn't sacrifice flavor or satisfaction.

Now, in 2024,I have compiled your favorite breakfast recipes into a comprehensive cookbook titled "Diabetes Breakfast Recipes Cookbook 2024." Through this book, My aim is to share my knowledge and experiences with others who are looking for healthy and delicious breakfast options that are suitable for diabetes management. With easy-to-follow recipes and practical tips, My cookbook is a valuable resource for anyone looking to start their day on the right foot while managing their diabetes.
You are going to enjoy this book, watch out for the bonus package at the end of this book. No rush. Here we go !

CHAPTER 1

UNDERSTANDING DIABETES

Diabetes is a complex disease that affects millions of people worldwide, with both Type 1 and Type 2 diabetes posing significant challenges. Type 1 diabetes occurs when the body stops producing insulin, requiring daily injections for survival. Type 2 diabetes, on the other hand, develops gradually as the body becomes less sensitive to insulin over time. Gestational diabetes, which affects women during pregnancy, can lead to dangerous conditions like preeclampsia and increase the risk of Type 2 diabetes in both mothers and children.

Understanding the root causes of diabetes is crucial for effective prevention and management. Factors such as stress, chronic depression, racism, and poverty are closely tied to diabetes. A holistic approach that considers these social determinants, along with dietary choices, genetic makeup, and exercise habits, can provide valuable insights into diabetes prevention and management.

Natural dietary methods, such as reducing sugar and refined carbohydrates and incorporating whole foods with healthy fats, have been shown to prevent and even reverse Type 2 diabetes. Intermittent fasting and carbohydrate-reduced diets can also be effective in managing diabetes.

CHAPTER 2

BUILDING A HEALTHY

DIABETES-FRIENDLY BREAKFAST

Building a healthy diabetes-friendly breakfast involves consuming a balanced meal that contains fiber-rich carbohydrates, protein, and healthy fats. This combination helps combat high morning blood sugar and keeps blood sugar levels steady. Traditional breakfast foods like bagels, doughnuts, pastries, pancakes, and French toast are often high in refined carbohydrates and sugar, which can cause blood sugar levels to spike. Instead, aim for a breakfast with protein, fiber-rich carbohydrates, and healthy fat. A dietitian's favorite breakfast for diabetes is Overnight Chia Oats, which contains 15 grams of protein, fiber-rich carbohydrates, and healthy fats. Physical activity also plays a huge role in blood sugar management, as our muscles' preferred source of fuel is glucose. Therefore, regular exercise can help use up glucose in the bloodstream. For the best blood-sugar-friendly breakfast, aim for a mix of fiber-rich carbohydrates, like whole grains, plus protein and healthy fats.

Importance of a Balanced Breakfast

A balanced breakfast is crucial for overall health and well-being. It supports brain function, improves concentration, and helps manage weight effectively. By kickstarting metabolism, breakfast boosts energy levels and enhances physical and mental performance. A nutritious breakfast can aid in heart health, weight management, and even contribute to better hair health. Including a variety of food groups like whole grains, proteins, fruits, and dairy ensures a well-rounded meal that provides essential nutrients for a productive day ahead.

Key Nutrients for Diabetes

Key nutrients for diabetes management include a balance of carbohydrates, protein, fats, vitamins, and minerals. Carbohydrates should come from whole, minimally processed sources such as vegetables, fruits, whole grains, and legumes.Fiber-rich foods can help regulate blood sugar levels and promote satiety. Protein is essential for growth, repair, and maintaining lean muscle mass; however, those with diabetic kidney disease should limit protein intake. Healthy fats, such as those found in nuts, seeds, avocados, and fish, can help reduce inflammation and support heart health. Vitamins and minerals, including magnesium, chromium, and omega-3 fatty acids, have been shown to improve insulin sensitivity and glucose metabolism. Limiting intake of saturated and trans fats, as well as added sugars and sodium, is also crucial for overall health and diabetes management. A plant-based diet has been shown to have a positive effect on both the prevention and treatment of type 2 diabetes, particularly for weight loss and blood sugar control. It is recommended to consult with a dietitian to develop an individualized eating plan based on current eating patterns and health goals.

Here are some key nutrients to add to your meals

1. Fiber:

Fiber can help regulate blood sugar levels and improve insulin sensitivity. Good sources of fiber include fruits, vegetables, whole grains, and legumes.

2. Protein:

Protein can help keep you feeling full and satisfied, which can help with weight management. Good sources of protein include lean meats, poultry, fish, tofu, beans, and nuts.

3. Healthy fats:

Healthy fats, such as monounsaturated and polyunsaturated fats, can help improve insulin sensitivity and reduce the risk of heart disease. Good sources of healthy fats include avocados, olives, nuts, seeds, and fatty fish.

4. Vitamins and minerals:

Certain vitamins and minerals, such as vitamin D, calcium, magnesium, and chromium, may help improve insulin sensitivity and blood sugar control.

5. Omega-3 fatty acids:

Omega-3 fatty acids, which are found in fatty fish, walnuts, and flaxseed, can help reduce inflammation and improve heart health.

6. Antioxidants:
Antioxidants, such as vitamins C and E, can help protect against cell damage and reduce the risk of complications.

7. Water:
Staying hydrated is important for overall health and can help regulate blood sugar levels. Aim to drink at least 8 glasses of water a day.

It's important to note that while these nutrients can be beneficial for diabetes management, they should also be part of a balanced diet and not used as a substitute for medical treatment. Take your medications as well. It's very important.

Recommended Serving Sizes

Recommended serving sizes are essential for maintaining a healthy diet and ensuring that you consume the right amount of nutrients. The American Heart Association recommends consuming 6 ounces of grains per day, with serving sizes including ½ cup cooked rice, pasta, or cereal, 1 oz. dry pasta or rice, 1 slice bread, or 1 cup ready-to-eat cereal flakes. The Dietary Guidelines for Americans, 2020-2025 recommend consuming 2 ½ cups of vegetables, 2 cups of fruits, 5 ½ oz. of protein foods, and 3 cups of fat-free or low-fat dairy foods per day.

It is crucial to understand the difference between a portion and a serving size. A portion is the amount of food you choose to eat at one time, while a serving size is the amount of food listed on a product's Nutrition Facts label.To manage portion sizes, it is recommended to check the nutrition facts label, serve the correct portion, eat from smaller dishes, and not go back for seconds. At a restaurant, one can ask about half portions, share an entrée, or choose a healthy appetizer instead of an entrée.

Recommended serving sizes are essential for maintaining a healthy diet and ensuring that you consume the right amount of nutrients. Understanding the difference between a portion and a serving size and managing portion sizes at home and when eating out will help you maintain a healthy weight and reduce the risk of chronic diseases.

Tips for Controlling Carbohydrates

To control carbohydrates effectively, consider these tips:

1.Choose Healthier Carbohydrates

Opt for whole grains, fruits, vegetables, legumes, and dairy products like unsweetened yogurt and milk. Avoid low-fiber foods like white bread and highly processed cereals.

2. Monitor Portion Sizes

Be mindful of portion sizes to manage carb intake accurately, especially when carb counting. Portion sizes vary, so find what works best for you.

3. Reduce Salt Intake

Limit salt consumption to 6g per day to lower the risk of high blood pressure, heart diseases, and stroke. Cook from scratch and use herbs and spices for flavor instead of salt.

4. Limit Red and Processed Meat

Avoid excessive consumption of red and processed meats like ham, bacon, and sausages due to their links with heart issues and cancers.

5. Cut Down on Sugary Foods

Swap sugary drinks with water, plain milk, or unsweetened tea and coffee. Consider using low or zero-calorie sweeteners to manage blood glucose levels and weight effectively[3].

6. Choose Wisely

Opt for complex carbohydrates like whole grains and vegetables over simple carbs found in sugars and sweets. Complex carbs offer more nutritional value and help with energy levels and digestion[4].

7. **Balanced Diet**

Incorporate a variety of foods, including proteins like poultry, fish, eggs, legumes, nuts, and seeds, to maintain a balanced diet while managing carb intake

By following these tips, you can effectively control your carbohydrate intake, manage blood glucose levels, and make healthier food choices to support your overall well-being.

CHAPTER 3

QUICK AND EASY DIABETES BREAKFAST RECIPES

Blueberry Oatmeal Bowl

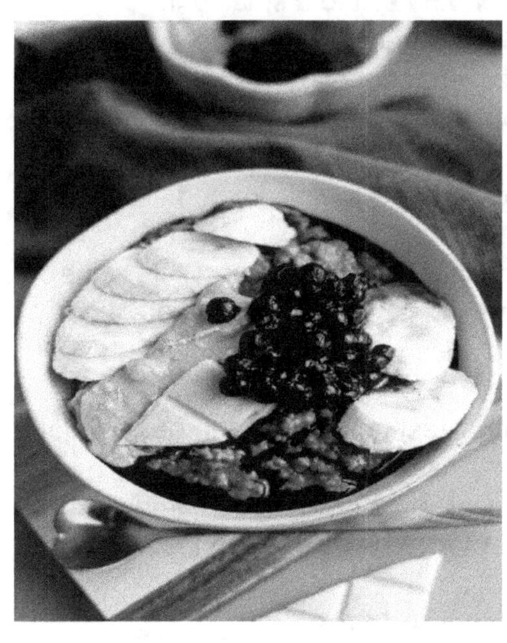

INGREDIENTS

- ½ cup milk of choice
- ½ cup water
- a pinch of salt
- ½ cup rolled oats
- ½ cup blueberries (fresh or frozen)
- ½ teaspoon lemon zest
- 2-4 teaspoons pure maple syrup

INSTRUCTIONS

- Add milk, water, and salt to a small pot.
- Stir everything together.
- Place the uncovered pot over medium-high heat until it starts to boil (it will take roughly 3 minutes to boil).
- Once the mixture starts to boil, immediately turn the heat down to low.
- Simmer the oatmeal for five minutes, this is the stage that hydrates the oats and gets them nice and soft (but not mushy!) and then remove the pot from the heat.
- Stir in the lemon zest and the blueberries and let it sit in the pot for a few minutes.
- Pour the oatmeal into a bowl, add the maple syrup, any other toppings you like and enjoy!

Optional Toppings/Add-ins

- Slivered almonds, walnuts, or pecans
- Shredded coconut
- Coconut yogurt
- Peanut butter or almond butter
- Strawberry sauce, blueberry compote, cherry sauce, or raspberry sauce
- More blueberries
- Chia seeds or ground flax seeds
- Pumpkin seeds or sunflower seeds
- Pomegranate seeds
- Cubed apples
- Hemp hearts
- Vanilla extract or any other extract you think would work well with the oatmeal you're making

Veggie Scrambled Eggs

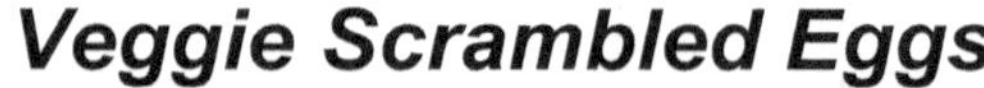

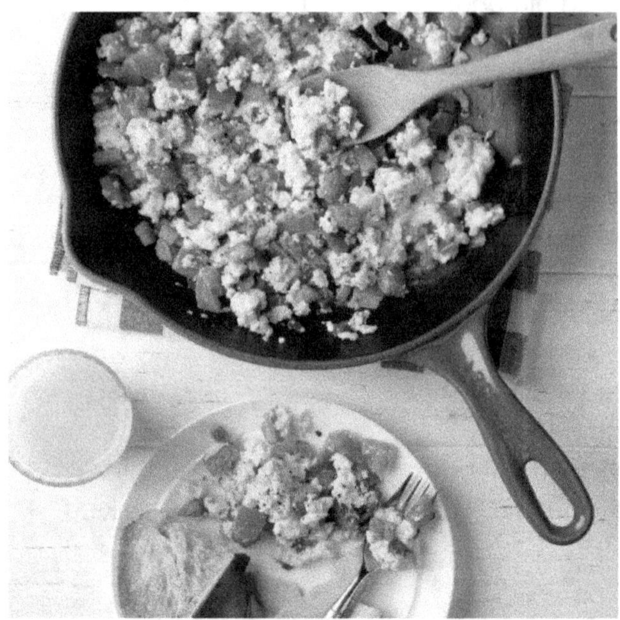

INGREDIENTS

- 2 teaspoons extra-virgin olive oil or cooking oil of choice
- 1 cup diced mixed veggies such as zucchini, mushrooms, scallions and peppers
- 4 large eggs, lightly beaten
- 1/8 teaspoon salt or to taste
- Freshly ground pepper to taste
- Pinch of Salt-free seasoning, such as Mrs. Dash
- 3 tablespoon Parmesan cheese

INSTRUCTIONS

- Heat oil in a large non-stick skillet over medium-high heat.
- Add veggies and cook, stirring often until softened and browned in spots, 2 to 4 minutes.
- Beat eggs, salt, pepper and salt-free seasoning in a small mixing bowl until combined.
- Pour eggs over the veggies.
- Cook, gently folding the eggs back with a spatula and allowing the uncooked eggs to flow onto the surface of the skillet.
- Once the eggs are mostly set-up stir less frequently to allow larger chunks of egg to form curds.
- Cook until it is no longer wet-looking, 1 to 2 minutes total.
- Remove from the heat and sprinkle with Parmesan before serving.

Greek Yogurt Parfait

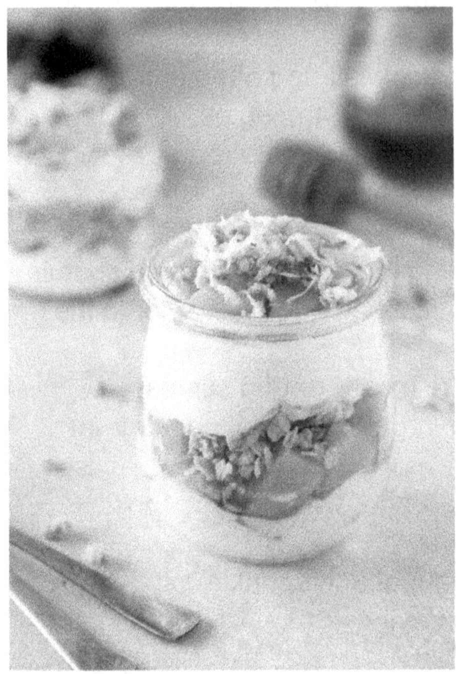

INGREDIENTS

- 1 tablespoon honey or maple syrup (optional)
- 3/4 cup plain Greek yogurt
- 1/4 cup berries or any other fruit cut into small 1-inch chunks
- 1/4 cup homemade granola or store-bought granola

INSTRUCTIONS

1. If using a sweetener, mix it with Greek yogurt in a small bowl until fully combined.
2. To layer the yogurt parfait, place half of the yogurt at the bottom of a mason jar or a bowl.
3. Top it off with half of the fruit and half of the granola.
4. Cover them with the rest of the yogurt and top it off with the rest of the fruit and granola.
5. If preferred, finish it off with a drizzle of honey.
6. Serve immediately.

Optional ingredients:
- A scoop of whey or plant-based protein powder
- A tablespoon of almond butter or peanut butter
- A handful of nuts and seeds
- Chocolate chips

Avocado Toast With Poached Eggs

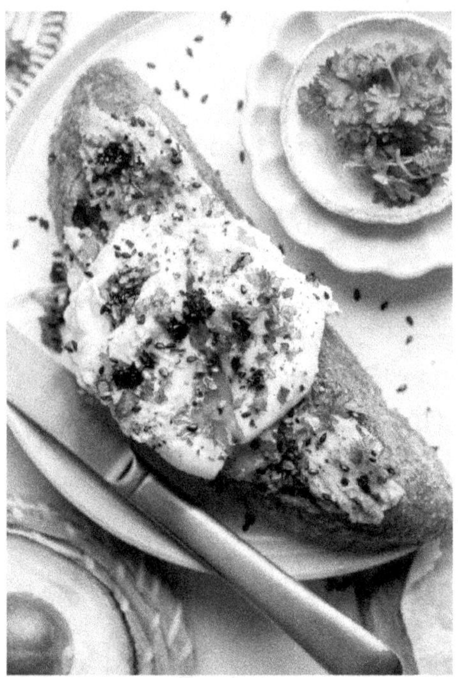

INGREDIENTS

- 2 eggs
- 2 slices whole grain bread
- 1/3 avocado
- 2 tablespoons shaved Parmesan cheese
- salt and pepper for topping
- fresh herbs for topping
- quartered heirloom tomatoes for serving

INSTRUCTIONS

- Bring a pot of water to boil.
- Drop the metal rims of two mason jar lids into the pot so they are laying flat on the bottom.
- When the water is boiling, turn off the heat and carefully crack the eggs directly into each rim.
- Cover the pot and poach for 5 minutes.
- While the eggs are cooking, toast the bread and smash the avocado on each piece of toast.
- When the eggs are done, use a spatula to lift the eggs out of the water.
- Gently pull the rim off of the eggs and place the poached eggs on top of the toast.
- Sprinkle with Parmesan cheese, salt, pepper, and fresh herbs; serve with the fresh quartered heirloom tomatoes.

Optional ingredients

- Sriracha or chili pepper flakes for a little heat
- Bacon
- A drizzle of balsamic reduction and olive oil
- Cheese (goat cheese or feta cheese work well)
- Smoked salmon, dill, and a squeeze of lemon
- Salsa or pico de gallo
- Pinto beans and a sprinkle of cumin
- Fresh mozzarella, tomatoes, and basil for a Caprese theme
- Roasted garlic-herb mushrooms pickled red onions and baby kale

Breakfast Smoothie Bowl

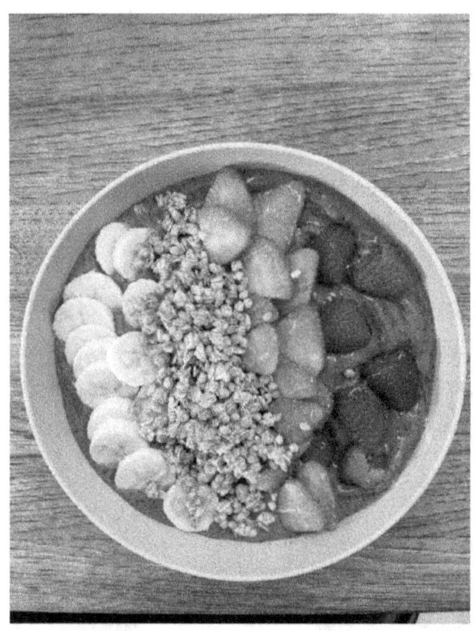

INGREDIENTS

- 1 ½ cups frozen mixed berries (or any frozen fruit)
- 1 banana (room temperature)
- ½ cup Greek yogurt
- ½ cup orange juice, plus more as needed
- Optional: 1 scoop protein powder or 1 tablespoon chia seeds
- Toppings: fresh berries, sliced bananas or other fruit, granola or nuts, coconut, almond butter, honey or maple syrup

INSTRUCTIONS

- Place the bowl for the smoothie in the freezer, then prepare the toppings (this helps to slow the melting process)
- Place the frozen fruit, banana, Greek yogurt and orange juice in a blender
- Blend until thick and smooth, adding a splash more orange juice as necessary
- Pour into the bowl and quickly top with the toppings
- Enjoy immediately

Note: For vegan, omit the Greek yogurt and add more orange juice until the smoothie blends. Consider adding the optional protein powder or chia seeds.

Mediterranean Spinach And Feta Frittata

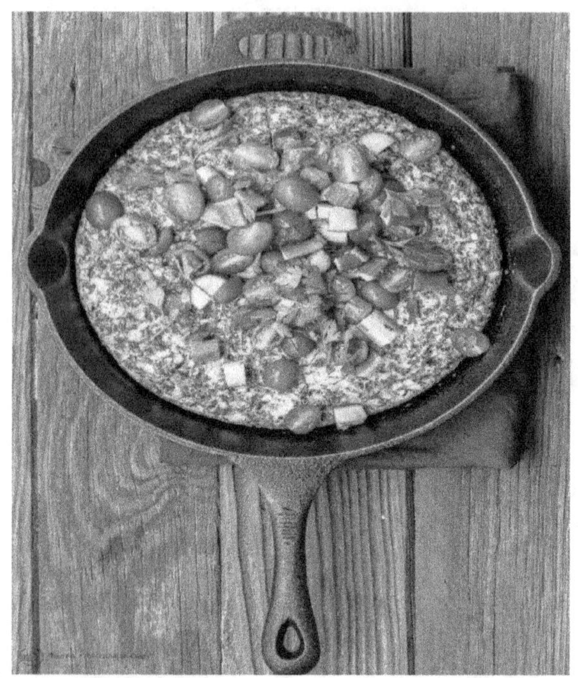

INGREDIENTS

- 1 tablespoon olive oil (extra virgin)
- 5 green onions
- 5 ounces baby spinach
- 3 ounces feta cheese
- 8 large eggs
- 4 egg whites

- 1/3 cup milk

- 1/2 cup cherry tomatoes
- salt and pepper to taste

INSTRUCTIONS

- Wash the green onions, chop the heads off, peel one layer, and then chop them into small pieces
- Roughly chop the spinach and set aside as well
- Cut the cherry tomatoes in half
- If using campari tomatoes, slice in round thin slices
- Crumble the feta cheese with your hands or with a fork and set aside
- Pre-heat the oven to 350 degrees Fahrenheit
- Add eggs to a bowl and whisk them
- Then add egg whites, milk, salt, pepper, and whisk again
- Place cast iron skillet on medium heat
- Once skillet is hot, add olive oil
- Then throw the green onions in
- Stir to saute them lightly
- Add spinach slowly and let it wilt, stir occasionally to turn it over
- Volume will go down fast
- Let the liquid coming out from spinach evaporate
- Pour whisked eggs over and add feta cheese all over the skillet
- Try to spread the cheese evenly
- The sides of the frittata will start to set but the middle should be all liquid still

- Insert a spatula on the sides to let more of the egg mix to flow underneath without breaking the frittata shape
- Add the cherry tomatoes halves on top, spread them around evenly
- After it's cooked for a few minutes, transfer cast iron skillet to oven and let cook for another 8 to 10 minutes until the middle of the skillet is not jiggly anymore
- Get the frittata out of the oven
- Make sure to not let it overcook
- Let it cool for a few minutes before cutting into it
- Usually, cut into 6 slices and serve with additional sides for breakfast/brunch or light meal

Quinoa Breakfast Porridge

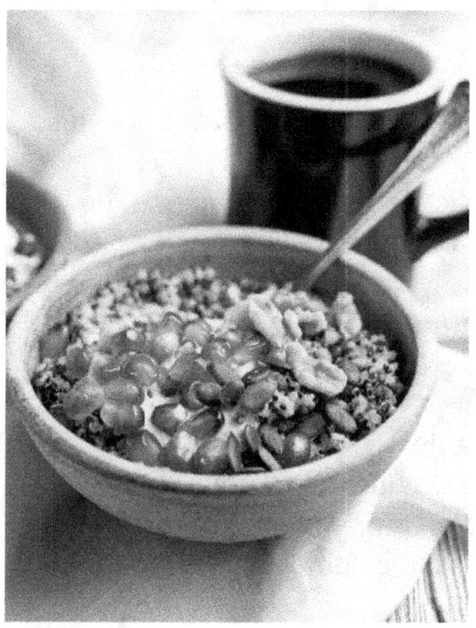

INGREDIENTS

- 1 cup of cooked quinoa
- ¼ cup uncooked
- 1 ½ cups (360 ml) of almond milk or your favorite milk
- ½ teaspoon of pure vanilla extract
- 1 teaspoon of maple syrup

Toppings

- Fresh fruit
- Nuts
- Seeds

- Peanut or almond butter

INSTRUCTIONS

1. Combine half a cup of quinoa with 1 cup or less of milk in a bowl.
2. Add vanilla extract and maple syrup and top with fresh fruit, seeds, and nuts and serve.

Nutrition Information:

This recipe provides approximate nutrition information for convenience and as a courtesy only. Nutrition data is gathered primarily from the USDA Food Composition Database. I get my research from the best before I prepare my meals so relax because you are in the safe hands of PAM J. RIOS.

Whole Wheat Pancakes With Berries

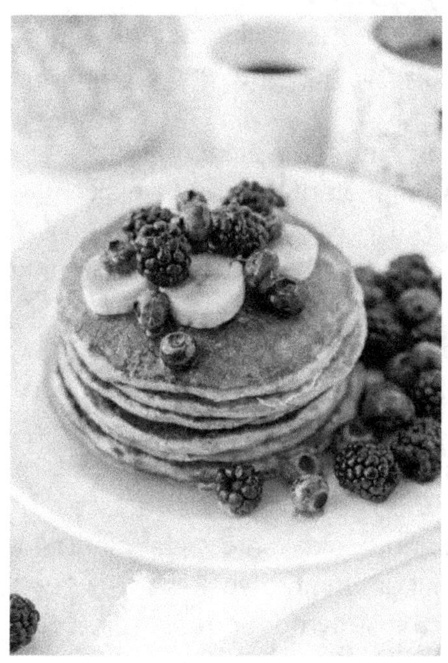

INGREDIENTS

- 1 cup whole wheat flour
- 2 tsp sugar
- 1/2 tsp baking powder
- 1/4 tsp baking soda
- 1/4 tsp salt
- 1 cup buttermilk
- 1 egg
- 2 tbsp melted butter
- 1 and 3/4 cups blueberries (fresh or frozen)
- Other berries of your choice (fresh or frozen)

INSTRUCTIONS

- In a large bowl, combine the dry ingredients (flour, sugar, baking powder, baking soda, and salt) and whisk together.
- In another bowl, combine the wet ingredients (buttermilk, egg, and melted butter) and whisk together.
- Whisk the wet mixture into the dry ingredients until just barely mixed. There should still be lumps.
- Fold in the blueberries and other berries.
- Preheat a nonstick griddle to 375 degrees F and grease the surface with butter.
- Add small scoops of pancake batter and cook for a few minutes until bubbles form on the surface.
- Flip the pancakes and cook for a couple minutes on the other side until golden brown.
- Serve with butter, maple syrup, or fresh fruit. Enjoy!

Overnight Chia Pudding

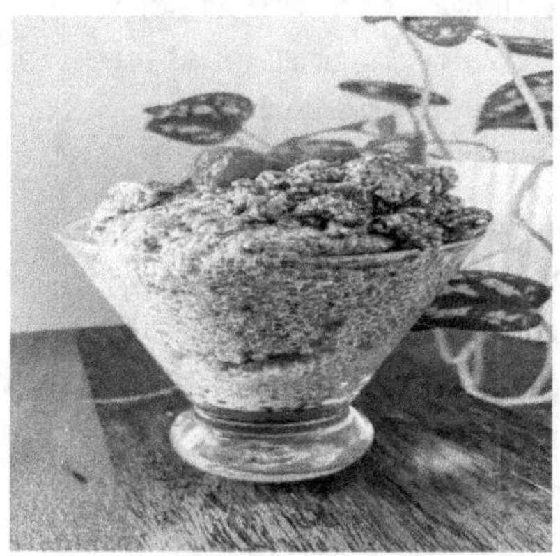

INGREDIENTS

- 1/4 cup cacao powder or unsweetened cocoa powder
- 3 to 5 tablespoons maple syrup
- 1/2 teaspoon ground cinnamon
- 1 pinch sea salt
- 1/2 teaspoon vanilla extract
- 1 1/2 cups unsweetened almond milk or light coconut milk
- 1/2 cup chia seeds

INSTRUCTIONS

- In a small bowl, combine the cacao powder, maple syrup, cinnamon, salt and vanilla extract. Whisk to combine.
- Add a little almond milk at a time and whisk until a paste forms.

- Add the remaining milk and whisk until smooth.
- Add chia seeds and whisk once more to combine.
- Cover and refrigerate overnight or at least three to five hours until it's achieved a pudding-like consistency.
- Give the mixture an extra whisk or stir once it has been in the refrigerator for 30 to 45 minutes.
- Leftovers can be kept covered in the fridge for four to five days, though best when fresh. Serve chilled with desired toppings, such as fruit, granola or coconut whipped cream.

TIPS

- Chia pudding is naturally gluten-free and can be switched to vegan, milk-free, dairy-free, paleo or keto.
- Chia seeds are a superfood, with lots of health benefits from minerals and antioxidants.
- Chia seeds are the richest plant source of omega-3s.
- Chia seeds are a good source of plant-based protein.
- Chia seeds are a good source of fiber.

Apple Cinnamon Breakfast Quinoa

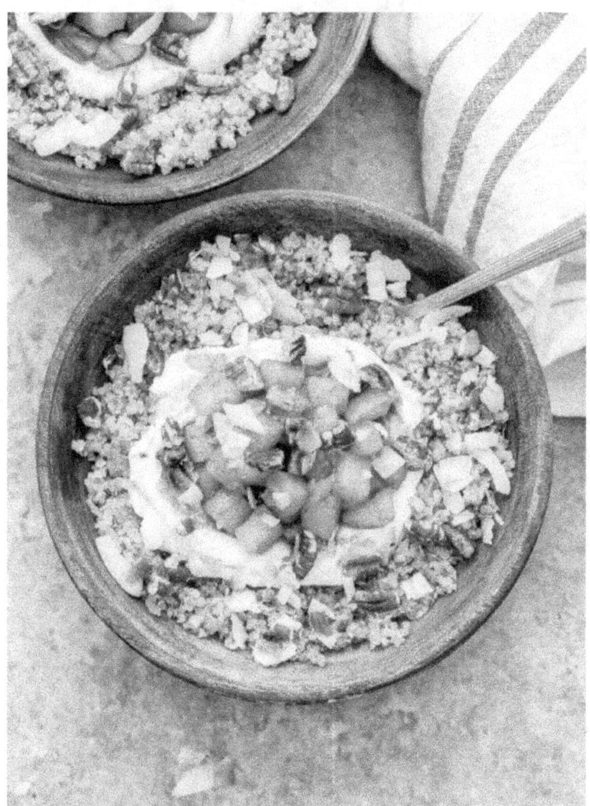

INGREDIENTS

- 1 cup of quinoa
- 2 cups of water
- 2 cups of diced apple
- 2 tablespoons of honey
- 1 teaspoon of cinnamon

- 1/4 cup of chopped pecans

INSTRUCTIONS

1. Combine quinoa, water, apple and cinnamon in a saucepan.
2. Bring to a boil, then reduce to a simmer for 20 minutes.
3. Stir in honey and pecans.
4. Serve warm.

Nutrition
Per serving: 340 calories, 8g fat, 63g carbs, 7g protein, 7g fiber, 30g sugar, 6mg sodium.

TIPS
- You can use any type of apple you like, but firmer apples like Granny Smith work best.
- You can also add other spices like nutmeg or ginger for extra flavor.
- This recipe makes a big batch, so feel free to halve the ingredients if you don't want leftovers.

- You can store leftovers in the fridge for up to 3 days or freeze for up to 2 months.

Enjoy!!

CHAPTER 4

HEARTY AND SATISFYING DIABETES BREAKFAST MEALS

Mushroom and Spinach Omelette

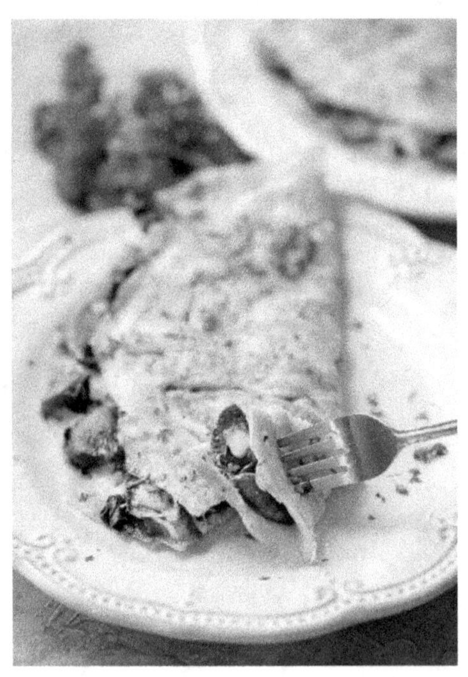

INGREDIENTS

- 2 Tbsp extra virgin olive oil
- 1 cup cremini mushrooms, thinly sliced
- 1 cup yellow onion, diced
- 1 cup fresh baby spinach
- 1/2 tsp kosher salt, divided
- 4 large eggs
- 1/2 tsp black pepper, divided
- 1/2 cup shredded Gruyere or Swiss cheese
- 2 Tbsp butter, divided
- Minced fresh parsley, for garnish
- Additional black pepper, for garnish
- Heat olive oil in a large skillet over medium-high heat

INSTRUCTION

- Add mushrooms and onion, cooking about 5 minutes, until golden and soft
- Season with 1/4 tsp salt and pepper, then stir in baby spinach until wilted
- Transfer mushroom mixture to plate and wipe out skillet
- Crack eggs into small mixing bowl with 1 Tbsp water and remaining salt and pepper, and beat with small whisk or fork until blended and a little frothy

- Add 1 Tbsp of butter to skillet and heat over medium to medium-low
- Add half of beaten egg mixture and stir them around the pan with a rubber spatula, pulling the sides in towards the middle, swirling the pan slightly so the runny egg mixture on top hits the pan and cooks
- Cook about 2 minutes, until eggs are just slightly shiny on top
- Add half of mushroom mixture to one side of the omelet, then sprinkle with 1/4 cup cheese
- Carefully lift up the edge of the omelet and check to see if the eggs are lightly golden on the bottom
- Once they are, gently fold it over the filling
- Slide omelet out of skillet and onto plate to serve
- Repeat steps 3 and 4 with remaining butter, egg mixture, mushroom mixture and cheese
- Serve garnished with minced parsley and extra black pepper if desired

Smoked Salmon Quiche

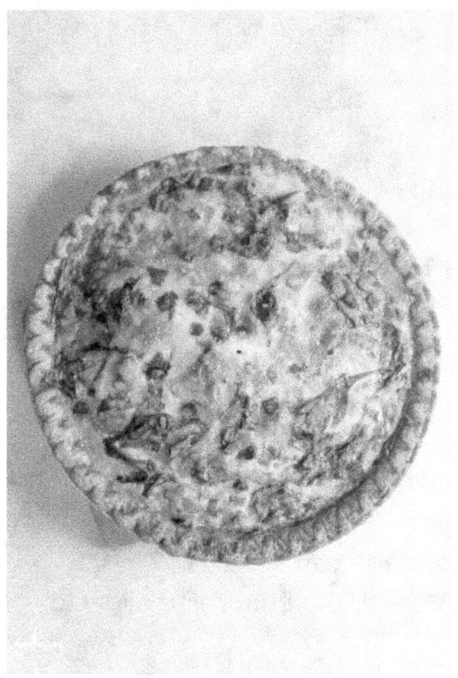

INGREDIENTS

- Crust:
    - 1 homemade quiche crust recipe (see notes)

- Filling:
    - 1 leek, thinly sliced (white part only)
    - 1/2 brown onion, thinly sliced
    - 2 garlic cloves, minced
    - 3/4 cup Gruyere cheese or cheddar, grated
    - 3 tbsp dill, finely chopped
    - 1 tbsp unsalted butter
    - 5 large eggs
    - 1 1/2 cups heavy cream
    - 1/2 tsp salt
    - 1 pinch pepper
    - 200 g smoked salmon (see notes)

INSTRUCTIONS

- Crust:
    - For the crust, you can either use a Perfect Quiche Crust Recipe or you can use 2 sheets of shortcrust pastry.
- Filling:
    - Preheat a fan forced oven to 320 F.
    - On medium heat, add the butter and allow to melt a little.
    - Next, add the sliced leek, onion and minced garlic. Stir for 2 minutes until they soften.
    - Don't let them brown. Take off the heat and allow to cool.
    - To a large mixing bowl or jug, add the eggs, cream, salt and pepper and 3/4 of the dill.
    - Whisk until well combined.

- Add the cooled leek mixture to the tart shell and spread around.
- Then add the smoked salmon ribbons.
- Sprinkle with cheese and pour on the egg mixture.
- Bake for 45 minutes or until golden and middle is still slightly jiggly.
- Allow to rest for 10 minutes before slicing.

NOTES

- Quiche can be stored in an airtight container in the fridge for up to three days.
- Quiche can be frozen in an airtight container or freezer bags for up to two months.
- You can use my recipe for Quiche Crust. It's flaky and buttery and so easy to make.
- But an alternative would be to use 2 sheets of frozen shortcrust pastry.
- Place two semi-thawed sheets of pastry on top of each other place on your workbench which has been dusted with flour.
- Roll out to about 12-inches in diameter.
- Use good quality smoked salmon for this recipe.

Mediterranean Breakfast Wrap

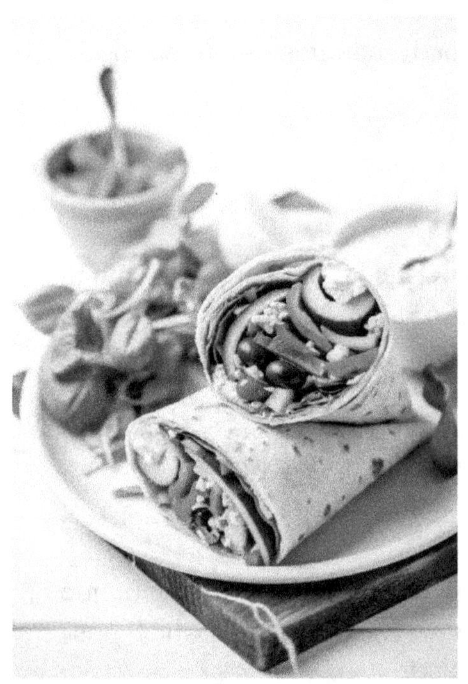

INGREDIENTS

- Whole grain or grain-free tortilla
- Hummus
- Egg and egg whites

- Onion
- Mushrooms
- Baby spinach
- Crumbled feta
- Sun-dried tomatoes
- Sea salt and pepper
- Hot sauce (optional)

INSTRUCTIONS

- Sauté vegetables in a skillet, onion and mushrooms for 3-4 minutes or until fragrant. Add spinach and sauté for a few minutes longer until spinach has wilted.
- Add egg and egg whites to pan with veggies and cook for about 2 minutes or until eggs are cooked through. Sprinkle on a little sea salt and ground pepper while cooking.
- Warm up the tortilla and spread on a layer of hummus. Place the egg scramble in the center of the tortilla and top with sun-dried tomatoes and feta. Sprinkle on a little more salt and pepper as well as hot sauce if using.
- Wrap tortilla up and serve!

Sweet Potato Hash with Eggs

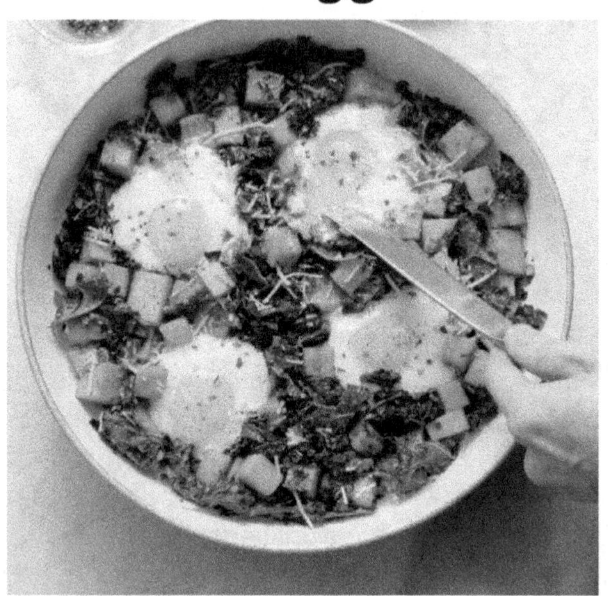

INGREDIENTS

- 2 tablespoons extra-virgin olive oil
- 1 cup red onion, ¼-inch dice
- 2 pounds sweet potato, washed, skin on, ½-inch dice
- ½ cup red bell pepper, ½-inch dice

- ½ cup green bell pepper, ½-inch dice
- 1 tablespoon minced garlic
- ¼ teaspoon smoked paprika
- sea salt, as needed for seasoning
- black pepper, as needed for seasoning
- 4 large eggs
- 1 tablespoon green onions, thinly sliced

INSTRUCTIONS

1. Preheat oven to 425°F.
2. Heat a large 10-inch ovenproof skillet like cast iron over medium heat.
3. Add 2 tablespoons olive oil, once hot add the red onions and saute for 1 minute.
4. Add garlic and saute for 1 minute.
5. Add sweet potatoes, ½ teaspoon salt and ¼ teaspoon black pepper, stir to combine and then allow the potatoes to cook unmoved to lightly brown the surface, 4 minutes. Stir and saute until tender, about 4 to 6 minutes.
6. Add bell peppers and saute for 2 minutes. Turn off heat, add smoked paprika and stir to combine.
7. Make four indents in the sweet potato to place the eggs in separate areas, leaving enough space in between.
8. Transfer pan to the oven and bake until the eggs just begin to set and the yolks still move when lightly shaking the pan, about 7 to 8 minutes.

9. Remove the pan from the oven and garnish with green onions and more salt and pepper as desired.

Breakfast Burrito with Turkey Sausage

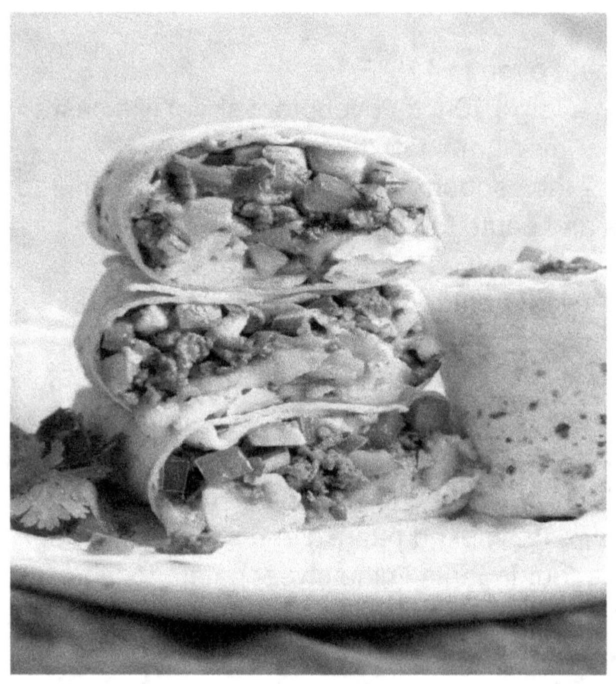

INGREDIENTS

- ½ lb (8 oz) uncooked 99% lean ground turkey breast
- ½ teaspoon salt, divided
- ¼ + ⅛ teaspoons black pepper, divided
- ⅓ teaspoon ground sage
- ⅓ teaspoon ground thyme
- ⅛ teaspoon dried marjoram
- ⅛ teaspoon crushed red pepper flakes
- ⅛ teaspoon paprika
- 4 large eggs
- 3 oz 50% reduced fat sharp cheddar cheese, divided
- ¼ cup salsa
- 1 tablespoon chopped fresh cilantro
- 4 low carb 8-inch tortillas

INSTRUCTIONS

- Place the ground turkey in a mixing bowl and add ¼ teaspoon of the salt, ¼ teaspoon of the black pepper, the sage, the thyme, the marjoram, the crushed red pepper, and the paprika.
- Mash/stir together with a fork or your hands until well combined.

- Mist a large skillet with cooking spray and bring over medium heat.
- Cook the seasoned ground turkey, breaking it up into small chunks, until cooked through.
- Transfer the cooked turkey into a clean mixing bowl.
- Wipe out the skillet with a paper towel.
- Combine the eggs and remaining ¼ teaspoon of salt and 1/8 teaspoon of black pepper and add a splash of water.
- Use a whisk to beat the eggs.
- Mist the skillet with cooking spray and bring over medium heat.
- Add the beaten eggs and cook, pushing them around with a spatula to scramble, for a few minutes until cooked through.
- Use the spatula to break the scrambled eggs up into small chunks.
- Transfer the eggs to the mixing bowl holding the turkey sausage.
- Add the shredded cheddar, salsa, and cilantro and stir to combine.
- Lay the tortillas on a clean, dry surface and divide the sausage and egg mixture amongst them (about 2/3 cup of filling on each tortilla).
- Fold in the edges of a tortilla and roll it up to make a wrap.
- Repeat with the remaining tortillas.
- Mist a griddle pan or large skillet with cooking spray and bring to medium heat.

- Place the rolled burritos onto the hot skillet seam-side-down and cook for 2-3 minutes until the bottoms are golden.
- Flip the burritos and cook for another 2 minutes until the other side is golden as well.

Coconut Flour Pancakes with Almond Butter

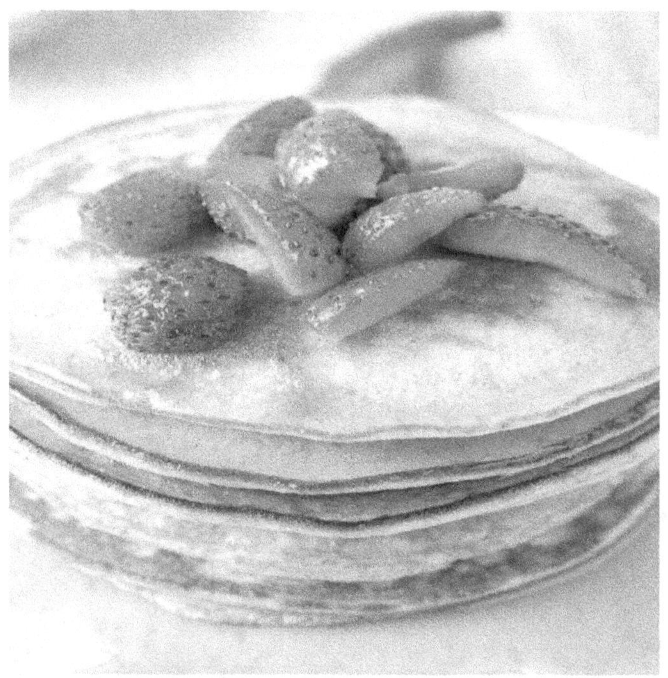

INGREDIENTS

For the pancakes:
- 1 cup spelt flour
- 1/2 cup coconut flour
- 3/4 tablespoon baking powder
- 1/2 teaspoon cinnamon

- 1/8 teaspoon nutmeg
- pinch of salt
- 1 1/2 cups milk of any kind (unsweetened if using nut milk)
- 1 egg
- 2 tablespoons melted coconut oil
- 2 tablespoons maple syrup
- 1/2 teaspoon vanilla

For the almond butter sauce:
- 1 tablespoon almond butter
- 1 tablespoon coconut butter
- 2-4 tablespoons milk of any kind

INSTRUCTIONS

For the pancakes:
1. Whisk together flours, baking powder, cinnamon, nutmeg and salt in a medium bowl.
2. Whisk together remaining wet ingredients in a small bowl.
3. Add the wet ingredients to the dry and stir until combined.
4. Heat a pancake griddle or pan over medium heat.
5. Grease your pan with desired fat and spoon batter in about 1/4 cup measurements onto pan forming a circular pancake shape.
6. Cook for about 2-3 minutes per side.

For the almond butter sauce:
1. Combine all ingredients in a small bowl.
2. Microwave for about 20 seconds.
3. Stir until creamy and smooth.

Breakfast Quesadilla with Black Beans

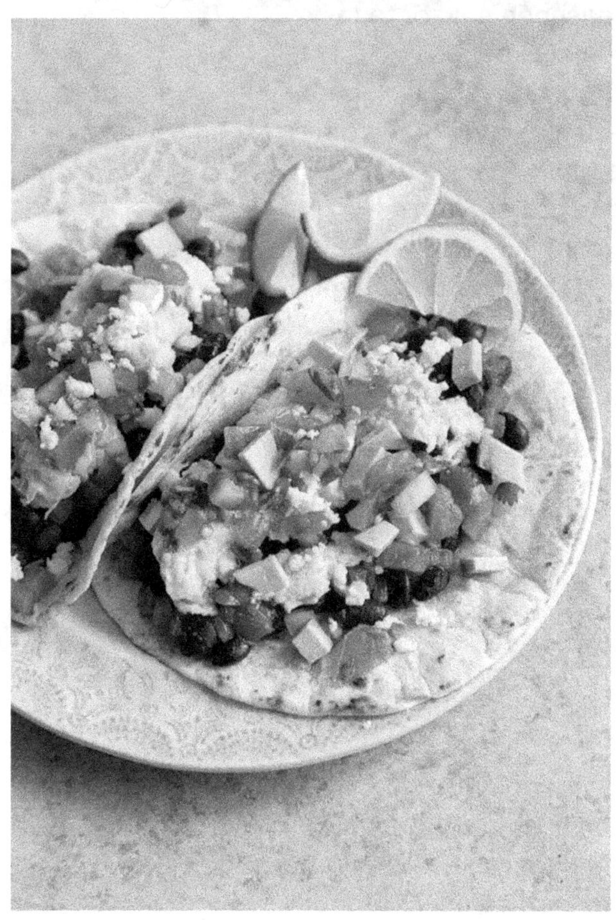

INGREDIENTS

- 2 teaspoons butter
- 1/4 cup red onion, chopped
- 6 large eggs, beaten in a bowl
- 1/8 teaspoon salt, or to taste
- Pinch black pepper
- 1 (15-ounce) can black beans, rinsed and drained
- 1 (4-ounce) can chopped mild green chiles,
drained
- 1/2 cup cilantro leaves
- 6 (9-inch) flour tortillas
- Pickled jalapeno peppers from a jar (optional)
- 1 1/2 cups grated sharp cheddar or Monterey jack
cheese, or more, to taste
- Vegetable oil, to reheat the quesadillas
- Salsa, to serve

INSTRUCTION

- Scramble the eggs:
In a nonstick skillet over medium heat, melt the
butter.
Add the onion and cook, stirring, for 30 to 40
seconds (just to soften them).
Add the eggs, salt, and pepper, and cook and stir
until they are set to your preference.
Remove the pan from the heat.
- Make the filling:

Stir the beans, mild green chiles, and cilantro into
the eggs in the pan.
- Assemble the quesadillas:
On one-half of each tortilla, spread about 1/2 cup of
the filling.
Top with a few jalapeno slices (if using) and 1/4 cup
cheese.
Fold and press together to flatten them.
- Cook the quesadillas:
Spray or brush a skillet with vegetable oil, then
place the skillet over medium heat.
Cook the quesadillas for 1 to 2 minutes on each
side, or until the cheese melts and the tortillas are
lightly browned and crisp on the outside.
- To serve:
Enjoy with salsa, if you like.

TO FREEZE:
Line a baking sheet that will fit in your freezer with
parchment paper or waxed paper.
Spread as many assembled quesadillas as will fit
on the baking sheet, top with a layer of paper, and
add a second layer.
Cover loosely with plastic wrap, and freeze until
firm, about 3 hours.
Transfer the frozen quesadillas to plastic freezer
bags, stacking them between small pieces of
parchment or waxed paper.
Store for up to 2 months.

TO REHEAT:

Remove as many quesadillas as you like from the freezer.

Spread on a microwave-safe plate and microwave for 2 minutes to partially defrost them.

At this point, the tortillas can be a little soggy, but that can be remedied.

Just follow the "Cook the Quesadilla" instructions in step.

Quinoa and Veggie Breakfast Bowl

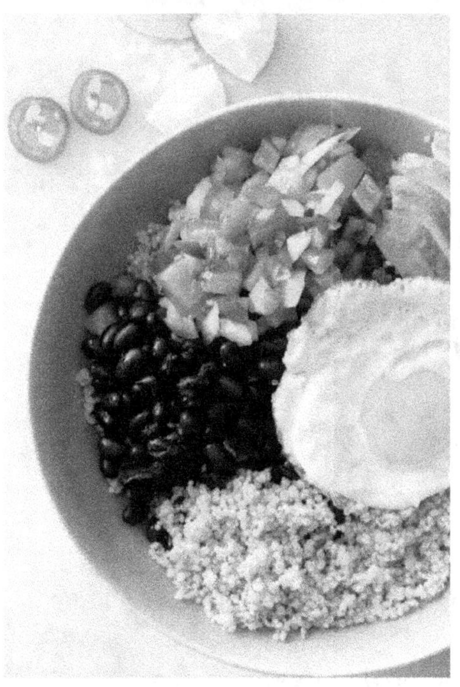

INGREDIENTS

- 1 cup cooked quinoa (about 1/3 cup dry)
- 2 cups kale chopped finely with the stems removed

- 1 tablespoon olive oil
- 1 tablespoon minced garlic
- 1/4 teaspoon salt
- 1/4 teaspoon pepper
- 1/2 avocado
- 4 eggs
- 1/2 batch dairy-free pesto

INSTRUCTION

Soft Boiled Eggs
1. Bring a small pot of water to a boil with 1/2 tsp baking soda.
2. Reduce the heat to low and add in the eggs.
3. Turn the heat back up to a boil and set a timer for 6 1/2 minutes.
4. Once the time is up, add the eggs into a bowl of ice water.
5. Crack the bottom of the egg onto a hard surface and peel off the rest of the shell.

Quinoa and Veggie Bowl
1. Sauté chopped kale in a pan with olive oil, garlic, salt and pepper for just a few minutes until the kale wilts.

2. Assemble your bowls with a base of quinoa and top with the kale, sliced avocado, the peeled eggs (sliced in half), pesto and red pepper flakes if desired.

Optional:
- Throw in some chopped tomatoes or mushrooms with the kale.
- Add a little hot sauce for spice.
- Use chickpeas instead of eggs for a vegan option.

Spinach and Mushroom Breakfast Casserole

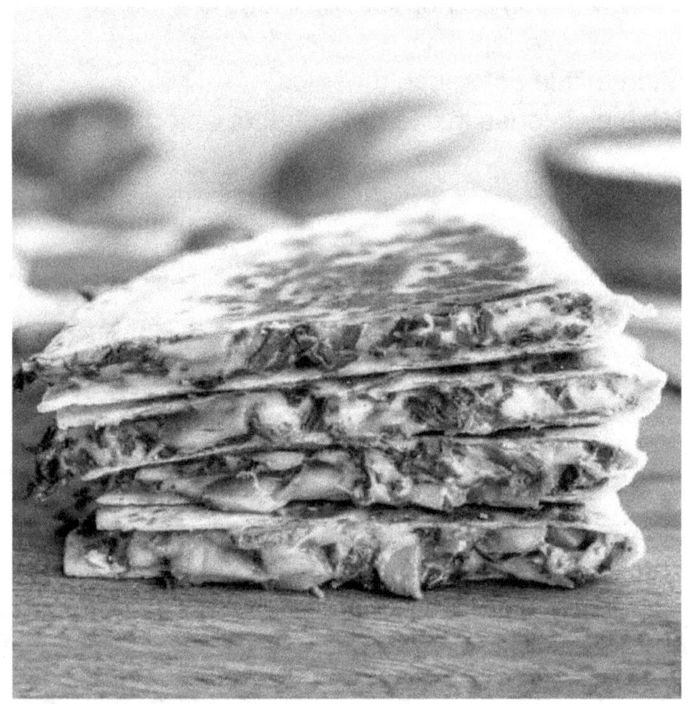

INGREDIENTS

- 1 lb. ground beef
- 1 cup minute rice (uncooked)

- 1 medium yellow onion (diced)
- 8 oz. mushrooms (chopped)
- 10.5 oz. cream of mushroom soup
- 1/2 cup sour cream
- 1 cup beef broth
- 1 sleeve Ritz crackers (crumbled)
- 1/4 cup butter (melted)

INSTRUCTION

- In a large skillet, brown the beef over medium-high heat with the onion and mushroom until the beef is no longer pink and the onions are translucent.
- Drain any fat, then transfer the beef mixture to a large casserole dish (9x13) mix in the mushroom soup, sour cream, rice, and beef broth. Combine well, and spread evenly in the dish.
- Spread cracker crumbs over the top of the casserole and drizzle with butter.
- Bake at 350°F for 30-40 minutes, uncovered, or until the rice is tender.

Zucchini and Parmesan Frittata

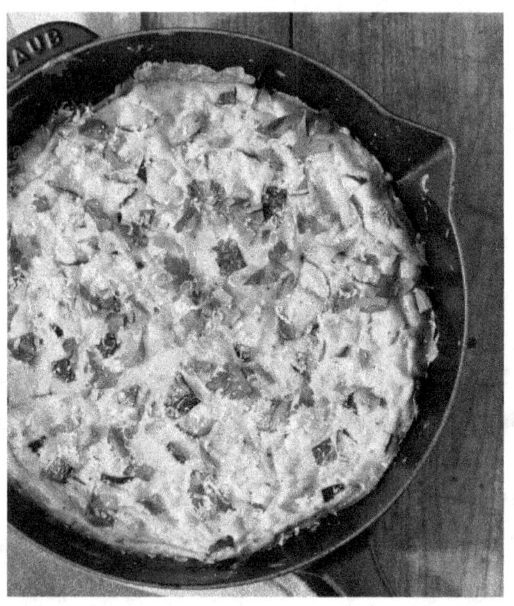

INGREDIENTS

- 6 large eggs
- 1 cup grated Parmesan cheese
- 1/2 cup thinly sliced zucchini
- 1/2 cup finely chopped onion
- 1 clove garlic, minced
- 2-3 tablespoons olive oil

- 1/2 teaspoon dried oregano
- Salt and pepper to taste

INSTRUCTIONS

1. *Prepare ingredients*: Grate the zucchini and squeeze out the excess moisture using paper towels. Whisk together eggs, milk, and spices.
2. *Sauté*: Cook garlic, onion, and zucchini in a cast-iron skillet for 8-10 minutes or until juices have cooked down from zucchini.
3. *Add eggs*: Pour the egg mixture into the pan, stirring everything together. Let cook 2 minutes or until edges begin to golden.
4. *Broil*: Sprinkle Parmesan cheese on top of eggs. Broil for 2-5 minutes or until the top is set and slightly browning.
5. *Serve*: Slice and serve while still warm. This tastes great on its own or with salsa, sour cream, plain yogurt, or hot sauce.

TIPS

- Use fresh Parmesan for the best flavor.
- Eggs cook fast, so there's no need to sauté them too long.
- Squeeze zucchini before cooking to remove excess moisture.

- Leftovers can be stored in an airtight container in the fridge for 3-4 days or frozen for up to 3 months. Just reheat in the oven or microwave to serve.

CHAPTER 5

DIABETIC-FRIENDLY BAKED GOODS AND TREATS

Almond Flour Banana Bread

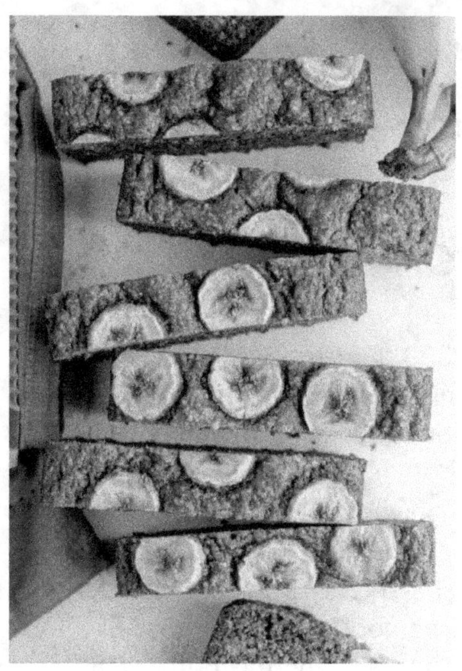

INGREDIENTS

- 3 medium-large very ripe bananas with brown spots (1 cup mashed)
- 3 large eggs
- 1/4 cup any sweetener (maple syrup, honey or sugar-free alternative)
- 1/4 cup any mild oil or melted butter (avocado oil, light olive oil, melted coconut oil or grapeseed oil)

- 1 teaspoon pure vanilla extract
- 1 teaspoon cinnamon
- 1 teaspoon baking soda
- 1 teaspoon baking powder
- 1/4 teaspoon salt
- 3 cups almond flour (not almond meal)
- Cooking spray (Misto)

INSTRUCTION

- Preheat oven to 350 degrees F. Line metal 9 x 5 loaf pan with parchment paper or leave non-stick as is. Spray only bottom and lower 1″ with cooking spray. Set aside.
- In a large mixing bowl, add bananas and mash with a masher. Then add eggs, sweetener, oil, vanilla, cinnamon, baking soda, baking powder and salt; whisk until combined.
- Add almond flour and stir and mix gently with spatula to combine.
- Pour batter into previously prepared loaf pan and bake for 50 minutes or until the toothpick inserted in the middle comes out clean.
- Remove almond flour banana bread from the oven and transfer to a cooling rack to cool off for 10 minutes. Remove bread from a loaf pan and let it cool off completely. Slice with sharp serrated knife.

Oatmeal Raisin Cookies

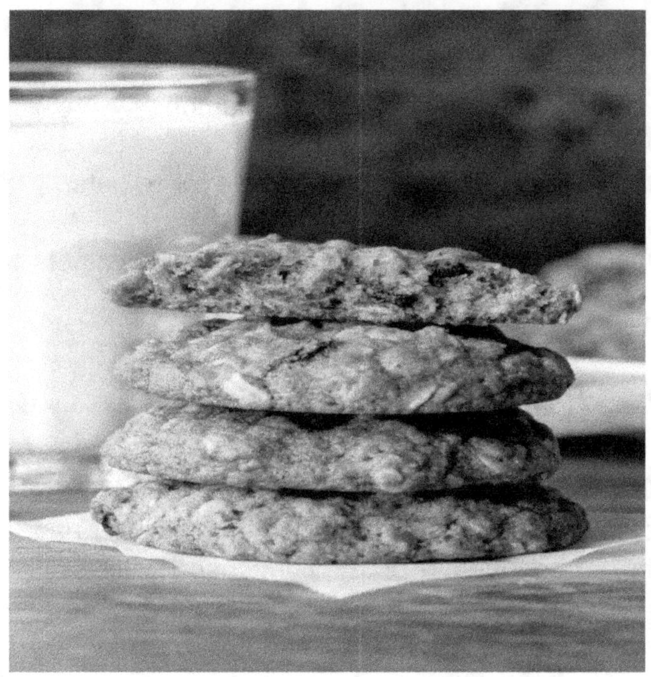

INGREDIENTS

- 1 cup (16 Tbsp; 226g) unsalted butter, softened to room temperature
- 1 cup (200g) packed light or dark brown sugar
- 1/4 cup (50g) granulated sugar
- 2 large eggs
- 1 Tablespoon pure vanilla extract

- 1 Tablespoon (15ml) unsulphured or dark molasses
- 1 and 1/2 cups (188g) all-purpose flour
- 1 teaspoon baking soda
- 1 and 1/2 teaspoons ground cinnamon
- 1/2 teaspoon salt
- 3 cups (255g) old-fashioned whole rolled oats
- 1 cup (140g) raisins
- Optional: 1/2 cup (64g) chopped toasted walnuts

INSTRUCTIONS

1. Using a hand mixer or a stand mixer fitted with paddle attachment, cream the softened butter and both sugars together on medium speed until smooth, about 2 minutes.
2. Add the eggs and mix on high until combined, about 1 minute.
3. Scrape down the sides and bottom of the bowl as needed.
4. Add the vanilla and molasses and mix on high until combined.
5. Set aside.
6. In a separate bowl, whisk the flour, baking soda, cinnamon, and salt together.
7. Add to the wet ingredients and mix on low until combined.
8. Beat in the oats, raisins, and walnuts (if using) on low speed.
9. Dough will be thick, yet very sticky.

10. Chill the dough for 30-60 minutes in the refrigerator (do the full hour if you're afraid of the cookies spreading too much).
11. If chilling for longer (up to 2 days), allow to sit at room temperature for at least 30 minutes before rolling and baking.
12. Preheat oven to 350°F (177°C).
13. Line two large baking sheets with parchment paper or silicone baking mats.
14. Set aside.
15. Roll balls of dough (about 2 tablespoons of dough per cookie) and place 2 inches apart on the baking sheets.
16. I recommend using a cookie scoop since the dough can be sticky.
17. Bake for 12-14 minutes until lightly browned on the sides.
18. The centers will look very soft and under-baked.
19. Remove from the oven and let cool on baking sheet for 5 minutes before transferring to a wire rack to cool completely.
20. The cookies will continue to "set" on the baking sheet during this time.

Banana Oat Muffins

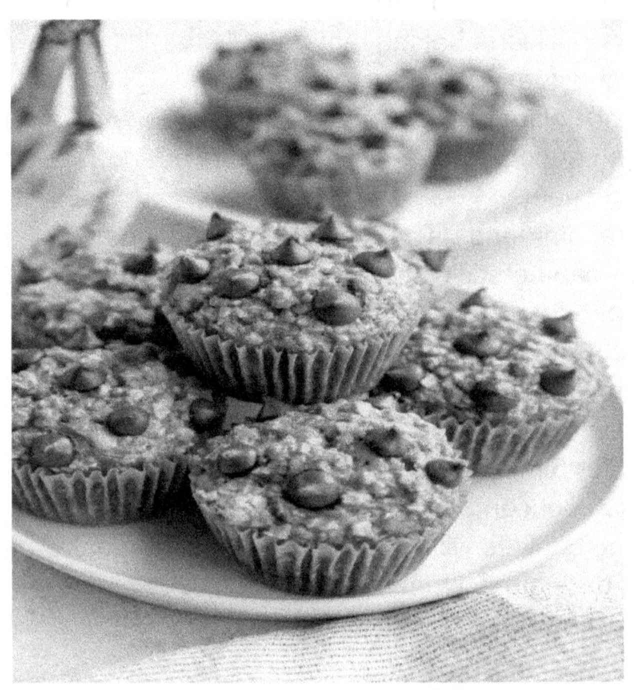

INGREDIENTS

Muffins:
- 1 large egg

- 1/4 cup oil
- 1 1/2 cups mashed banana
- 1 teaspoon vanilla extract
- 1 1/2 cups old-fashioned oats
- 1 1/4 cups all-purpose flour
- 1/4 cup granulated sugar
- 1/4 cup brown sugar
- 1 1/2 teaspoons baking powder
- 1 teaspoon baking soda
- 1/2 teaspoon cinnamon
- 1/4 teaspoon salt

Topping:
- 2/3 cup old-fashioned oats
- 3 tablespoons brown sugar
- 1 tablespoon all-purpose flour
- 1/4 teaspoon cinnamon
- 3 tablespoons butter melted

INSTRUCTION

1. Preheat oven to 375 F.
2. Grease or line a standard 12-cup muffin tin and set aside.
3. Whisk the egg and oil together in a large mixing bowl.
4. Add the mashed banana and vanilla extract.
5. Whisk in until well combined.

6. Add the oats, flour, sugars, baking powder, baking soda, cinnamon and salt.
7. Whisk in just until combined.
8. Divide the muffin batter between the prepared muffin tin cups.
9. To make the topping, stir the oats, sugar, flour and cinnamon together.
10. Mix in the melted butter until combined.
11. Divide the topping between the muffin tin cups and sprinkle over the batter.
12. Bake for 20 to 25 minutes, or until a toothpick inserted in the center of a muffin comes out clean.
13. Let cool in pan for 10 minutes.
14. Remove to a wire rack to finish cooling.

Carrot Cake Breakfast Bars

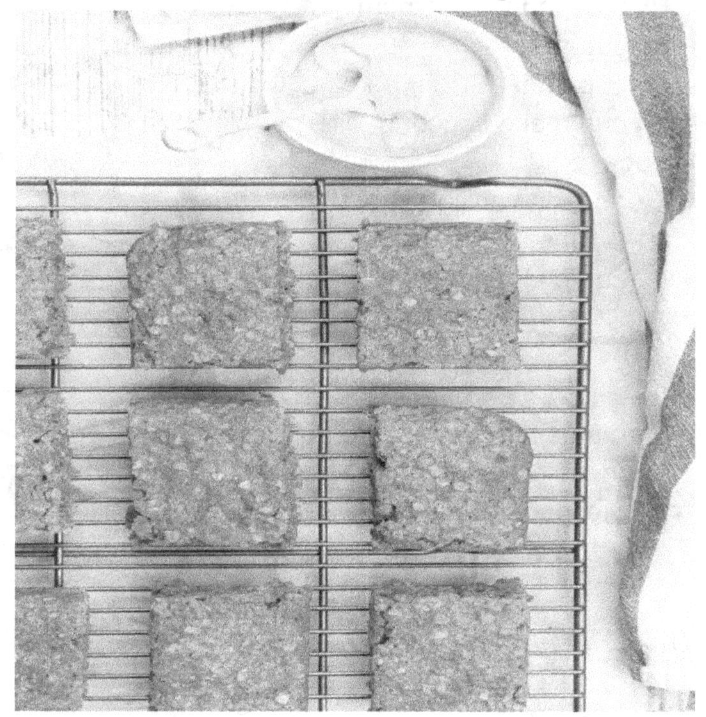

INGREDIENTS

- 1 1/2 cups regular oats
- 1 cup whole wheat flour
- 1/4 cup ground flaxseed
- 1 teaspoon cinnamon
- 1/2 teaspoon nutmeg

- 1/2 teaspoon baking powder
- 1/4 teaspoon ground allspice
- 1/4 teaspoon salt
- 1/8 teaspoon cardamom
- 3/4 cup milk
- 1/4 cup honey
- 1/4 cup melted coconut oil
- 1 egg
- 1 teaspoon vanilla extract
- 1 1/2 cups grated carrots
- 1/2 cup chopped walnuts (optional)

Ingredients for the honey cream cheese
- 8 ounces cream cheese
- 1 tablespoon honey

INSTRUCTIONS

1. Preheat the oven to 350 degrees Fahrenheit.
2. In a large bowl, combine the oats, flour, flaxseed, cinnamon, nutmeg, baking powder, allspice, salt, and cardamom.
3. In a separate bowl, combine the milk, honey, melted coconut oil, egg, and vanilla extract.
4. Add the wet ingredients to the dry ingredients and stir until combined.
5. Fold in the grated carrots and chopped walnuts (if using).

6. Press the mixture into a lined or greased 8x8-inch baking dish.
7. Bake for 25-30 minutes or until lightly golden brown.
8. Allow the bars to cool completely before cutting into bars.
9. For the drizzle, combine the cream cheese and honey in a bowl and mix until smooth.
10. Drizzle the cream cheese mixture over the cooled bars.
11. Store the bars in an airtight container in the fridge for up to 5 days.

Cinnamon Apple Crumble

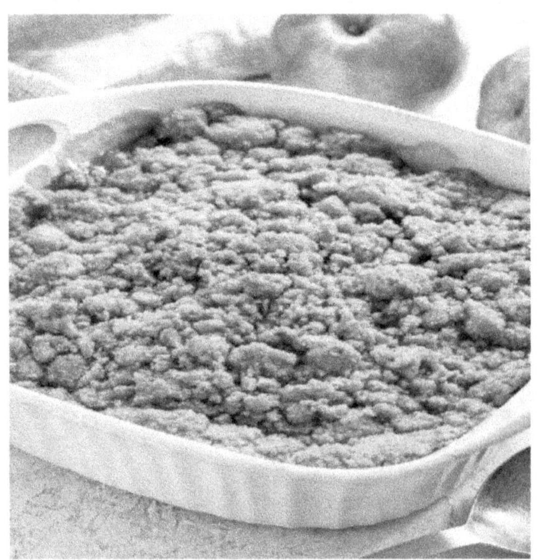

INGREDIENTS

For the apples:
- 6 Bramley apples
- 50 g caster sugar
- 2 teaspoon ground cinnamon
- 2 tablespoon water

For the crumble topping:

- 125 g plain flour
- 125 g rolled oats
- 125 g light brown sugar
- 125 g unsalted butter, melted

INSTRUCTIONS

1. Preheat the oven to 350 degrees Fahrenheit.
2. Make the crumble topping by pouring melted butter onto the flour, oats and light brown sugar. Mix with a spoon until crumbles form.
3. Peel and thinly slice the apples, and mix with the cinnamon, caster sugar, and water in a 2-liter pie dish.
4. Spoon over the crumble topping and bake in the oven for 35-45 minutes until golden and the fruit underneath is bubbling.
5. Allow to cool for 10 minutes before serving.

Top Tips:
- Don't skip the water for the apple filling. It helps to soften the apples so they become tender and fluffy.
- Don't forget the cinnamon either! Cinnamon pairs wonderfully with apples and adds a warm, comforting flavor to the crumble.
- As there is no pre-cooking of the apples in this recipe, slice the apples as thinly as you can, so they cook evenly and become soft and tender.

Variations:
- Add 1 peeled and sliced pear to the recipe for an apple and pear crumble.
- Add a handful of chopped walnuts to the crumble topping for added crunch and texture.
- Add a handful of dried cranberries or raisins to the apple filling for an extra fruity hit.
- Add half a teaspoon of ground ginger to the apple filling for extra warmth and spice.

Storage:
- Leftovers can be stored in the fridge for up to 3 days.
- Reheat in the microwave, or eat at room temperature.
- The crumble is also suitable for freezing.

Blueberry Walnut Scones

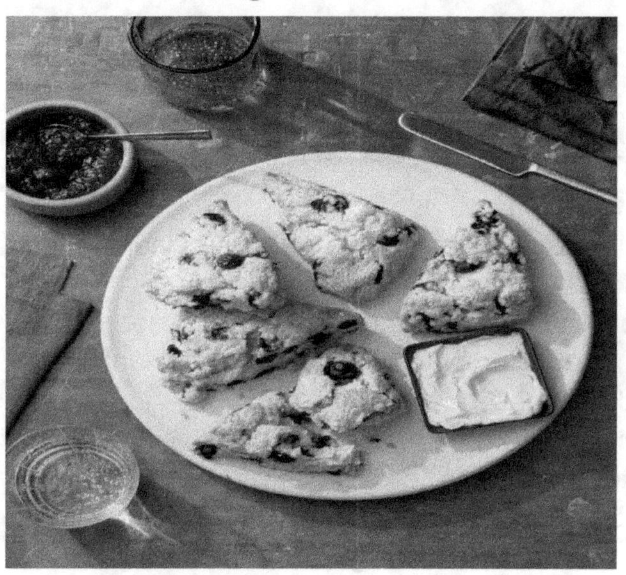

INGREDIENTS

- 2 cups all-purpose flour
- 1/2 cup granulated sugar
- 2 1/2 teaspoons baking powder
- 1 teaspoon ground cinnamon
- 1/2 teaspoon salt
- 1/2 cup unsalted butter, frozen
- 1/2 cup heavy cream
- 1 large egg
- 1 1/2 teaspoons pure vanilla extract
- 1 heaping cup fresh or frozen blueberries
- 1 cup chopped walnuts

INSTRUCTIONS

- Whisk flour, sugar, baking powder, cinnamon, and salt together in a large bowl
- Grate the frozen butter and add to the flour mixture and combine with a pastry cutter until pea-sized crumbs form
- Whisk heavy cream, egg, and vanilla extract together in a small bowl
- Drizzle over the flour mixture, add the blueberries and walnuts, then mix together until everything appears moistened
- Pour onto the counter and, with floured hands, work dough into a ball
- Press into an 8-inch disc and cut into 8 wedges
- Brush scones with remaining heavy cream and for extra crunch, sprinkle with coarse sugar
- Place scones on a plate or lined baking sheet and refrigerate for at least 15 minutes
- Preheat oven to 400 F
- Line a large baking sheet with parchment paper or silicone baking mat
- Arrange scones 2-3 inches apart on the prepared baking sheet
- Bake for 22-25 minutes or until golden brown around the edges and lightly browned on top

- Remove from the oven and cool for a few minutes before topping with vanilla icing

Pumpkin Spice Pancakes

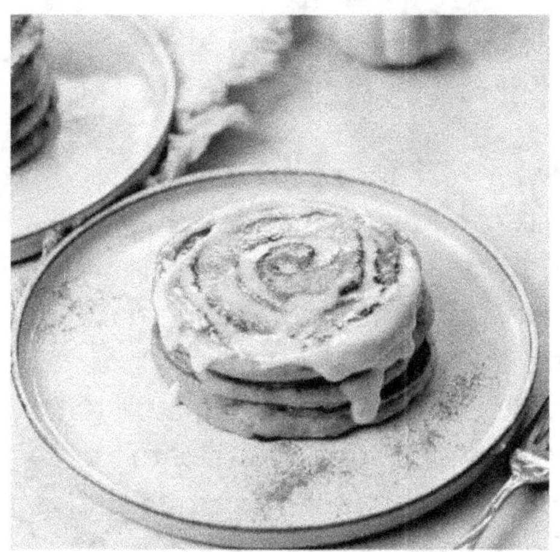

INGREDIENTS

- 2 cups all-purpose flour
- 3 tablespoons brown sugar
- 2 teaspoons baking powder
- 2 teaspoons cinnamon
- 2 teaspoons pumpkin pie spice
- 1/2 teaspoon salt
- 2 large eggs
- 3/4 cup pumpkin puree

- 3/4 cup milk of choice
- 1/4 cup neutral oil

INSTRUCTION

- In a medium bowl, combine the flour, brown sugar, baking powder, cinnamon, pumpkin pie spice, and salt.
- In a separate bowl, whisk together the eggs, pumpkin puree, milk, and oil (or melted butter).
- Stir the wet ingredients into the dry ingredients and mix with a spatula until no dry patches remain and a smooth batter forms.
- Lightly butter a skillet or griddle and wipe off extra grease with a paper towel. Heat the skillet to medium-low heat. Pour the batter into small circles (about 1/4 cup). Cook the pancakes until the bubbles pop on the top and the bottoms are golden. Then flip them and cook until cooked through and no longer gooey at the edges.
- Place the cooked pancakes under an inverted bowl to keep them warm. Repeat with the remaining batter, adjusting the heat as necessary to maintain an even temperature. Serve immediately with butter and maple syrup.

Enjoy your delicious Pumpkin Spice Pancakes!

Chocolate Avocado Brownies

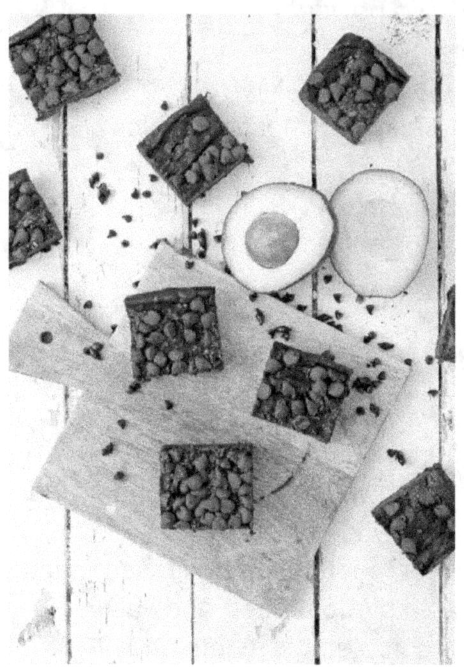

INGREDIENTS

- 1 large avocado peeled and pitted
- 2 large eggs at room temperature
- 1/3 cup coconut sugar or light brown sugar
- 1/4 cup pure maple syrup

- 3 tablespoons unsalted butter at room temperature
- 1 teaspoon pure vanilla extract
- 1/2 cup plus 2 tablespoons unsweetened cocoa powder
- 1/2 cup blanched almond flour
- 1 teaspoon espresso powder
- 1 teaspoon baking soda
- 1/2 teaspoon kosher salt
- 1/2 cup dark or semisweet chocolate chips

INSTRUCTIONS

1. Preheat the oven to 350 degrees F.
2. Line an 8x8-inch pan with parchment paper and coat with nonstick spray.
3. In a food processor, combine the avocado, eggs, coconut sugar, maple syrup, butter, and vanilla.
4. Process until it's completely smooth and combined.
5. Add the cocoa powder, almond flour, espresso powder, baking soda, and salt.
6. Process until smooth.
7. Add 1/4 cup chocolate chips and pulse a few times until roughly incorporated.

8. Scrape the batter into the prepared pan, smooth the top and sprinkle over the remaining 1/4 cup chocolate chips.

9. Bake for 25 to 30 minutes, until the top is set and a toothpick inserted in the center comes out mostly clean with just a few moist crumbs clinging to it.

10. Place the pan on a wire cooling rack and let the brownies cool for 30 minutes.

11. With the parchment paper handles, lift the brownies from the pan and place them on the rack to cool completely.

12. If time allows, refrigerate for at least 4 hours or overnight.

13. Slice and serve.

Raspberry Almond Oat Bars

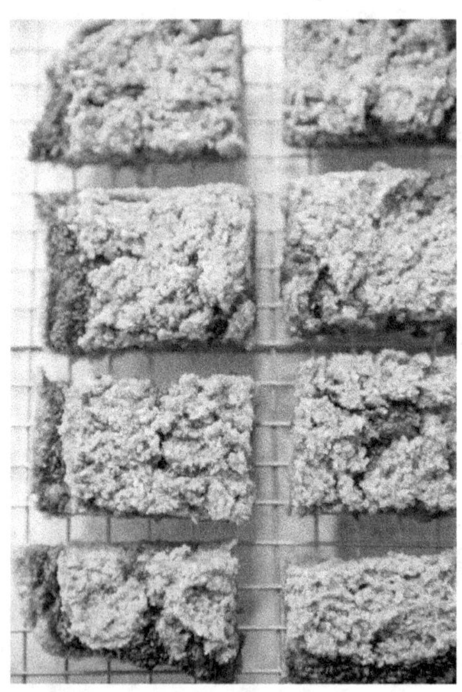

INGREDIENTS

Crust and Crumble:
- 2 cups almond flour
- 1 cup rolled oats

- 1 tsp baking powder
- 1/2 tsp salt
- 1/2 cup maple syrup
- 1/2 cup almond butter

Filling:
- 2 cups fresh raspberries
- 1 tbsp maple syrup

INSTRUCTIONS

- Preheat oven to 350F and line an 8x8 baking pan with parchment paper or nonstick spray.
- Mash raspberries and maple syrup together and set aside.
- In a large bowl, combine almond flour, oats, baking powder and salt.
- Add in maple syrup and almond butter and stir until everything is well combined.
- Save a 1 cup of dough to the side and flatten the rest into the 8x8 dish, pressing down firmly on the bottom.
- Pour raspberry mixture over top of uncooked crust.
- Crumble the remainder of the dough evenly over top of filling and bake for 40-45 minutes or until golden brown.

- Let cool before cutting. Store in fridge.

Lemon Poppy Seed Muffins

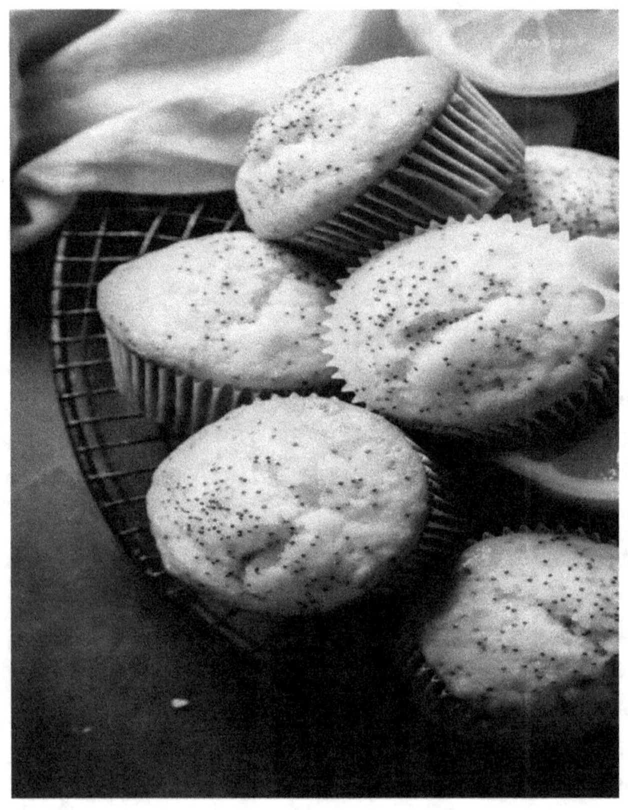

INGREDIENTS

- 1 3/4 cups all-rpose flour
- 1 teaspoon baking powder
- 1 teaspoon baking soda
- 1/2 teaspoon salt
- 2 tablespoons poppy seeds
- 1/2 cup unsalted butter, softened
- 1/2 cup granulated sugar
- 1/4 cup packed light or dark brown sugar
- 2 large eggs
- 1/2 cup sour cream or plain yogurt
- 1 1/2 tablespoons fresh lemon zest
- 3 tablespoons fresh lemon juice
- 1 1/2 teaspoons pure vanilla extract
- 1/4 cup milk

Lemon Icing:
- 1 cup confectioners' sugar, sifted
- 1 1/2 tablespoons lemon juice
- 1 tablespoon milk

INSTRUCTIONS

1. Preheat oven to 425 degrees Fahrenheit. Spray a 12-count muffin pan with nonstick spray or line with cupcake liners. Set aside.

2. In a large bowl, whisk the flour, baking powder, baking soda, salt and poppy seeds together. Set aside.

3. In a large bowl using a handheld or stand mixer fitted with a paddle attachment, beat the butter, sugar and brown sugar together on high speed until smooth and creamy, about two minutes. Scrape down the sides and bottom of the bowl as needed. Add the eggs, sour cream, vanilla extract, lemon zest and lemon juice. Beat on medium speed for one minute, then turn up to high speed and beat until combined. Scrape down the sides and bottom of the bowl as needed. Mixture may look a little chunky and curdled; that's okay.

4. With the mixer running on low speed, add the dry ingredients and milk into the wet ingredients and beat until no flour pockets remain.

5. Spoon the batter evenly into each muffin cup or liner. Bake the muffins for five minutes at 425 degrees Fahrenheit, then, keeping the muffins in the oven, reduce the oven temperature to 350 degrees Fahrenheit. Bake for an additional 15 to 17 minutes or until a toothpick inserted in the center comes out clean. The total time these muffins take in the oven is about 20 to 22 minutes. Allow the muffins to cool for five minutes in the muffin pan, then transfer to a wire rack to continue cooling.

6. Make the icing: Whisk all of the icing ingredients together and drizzle over warm or cooled muffins.

7. Cover and store leftover muffins for up to three days at room temperature or up to one week in the refrigerator.

CHAPTER 6

SAMPLE MEAL PLANS FOR DIABETES-FRIENDLY BREAKFASTS

Seven-Day Meal Plan

Here is my personal seven days meal Plan, it's all yours. Follow the Instructions to get the best meals. *Enjoy?*

Day 1
- *Breakfast:* 4 Egg Muffins (352 calories & 8 g carbs)
- *Snack:* 5.2 oz (148 g) Greek yogurt (0%) + 1 oz. (28 g) almonds (248 calories & 12 g carbs)

Day 2
- *Breakfast:* 4 Egg Muffins (352 calories & 8 g carbs)
- *Snack:* 4 oz. (114 g) apple + 1 tsp. nut butter (155 calories & 20 g carbs)

Day 3
- *Breakfast:* 1.5 serving Cauliflower Oatmeal + 2 eggs (353 calories & 25 g carbs)
- *Snack:* 4 oz. (114 gram) hummus (200 calories & 17 g carbs)

Day 4
- *Breakfast:* 1 serving Chia Seed Pudding (201 calories & 23 g carbs)
- *Snack:* 4 oz. (114 gram) apple + 1 tsp. nut butter (155 calories & 20 g carbs)

Day 5
- *Breakfast:* 1 serving Chia Seed Pudding + 2 eggs (345 calories & 24 g carbs)
- *Snack:* 5.2 oz (148 g) Greek yogurt (0%) + 1 oz. (29 g) almonds (248 calories & 12 g carbs)

Day 6
- *Breakfast:* 1 serving Protein Pancakes + 2 tsp. nut butter (372 calories & 24 g carbs)
- *Snack:* 1 serving Keto Peanut Butter Fat Bombs (247 calories & 3 g carbs)

Day 7
- *Breakfast:* 1 serving Cottage Cheese Pancakes + 1 tsp. nut butter (300 calories & 23 g carbs)
- *Snack:* 5 oz. (143 gram) Shelled edamame (200 calories & 14 g carbs)

Two-Week Meal Plan

Here is my personal Two weeks meal Plan.

Day 1-2
- *Breakfast:* 4 Egg Muffins (352 calories & 8 g carbs)
- *Snack:* 5.2 oz (148 g) Greek yogurt (0%) + 1 oz. (28 g) almonds (248 calories & 12 g carbs)

Day 3
- *Breakfast:* 1.5 serving Cauliflower Oatmeal + 2 eggs (353 calories & 25 g carbs)
- *Snack:* 4 oz. (114 gram) hummus (200 calories & 17 g carbs)

Day 4
- *Breakfast:* 1 serving Chia Seed Pudding (201 calories & 23 g carbs)
- *Snack:* 4 oz. (114 gram) apple + 1 tsp. nut butter (155 calories & 20 g carbs)

Day 5
- *Breakfast:* 1 serving Chia Seed Pudding + 2 eggs (345 calories & 24 g carbs)
- *Snack:* 5.2 oz (148 g) Greek yogurt (0%) + 1 oz. (29 g) almonds (248 calories & 12 g carbs)

Day 6

- *Breakfast:* 1 serving Protein Pancakes + 2 tsp. nut butter (372 calories & 24 g carbs)
- *Snack:* 1 serving Keto Peanut Butter Fat Bombs (247 calories & 3 g carbs)

Day 7
- *Breakfast:* 1 serving Cottage Cheese Pancakes + 1 tsp. nut butter (300 calories & 23 g carbs)
- *Snack:* 5 oz. (143 gram) Shelled edamame (200 calories & 14 g carbs)

Day 8-9
- *Breakfast:* 4 Egg Muffins (352 calories & 8 g carbs)
- *Snack:* 5.2 oz (148 g) Greek yogurt (0%) + 1 oz. (28 g) almonds (248 calories & 12 g carbs)

Day 10
- *Breakfast:* 1.5 serving Cauliflower Oatmeal + 2 eggs (353 calories & 25 g carbs)
- *Snack:* 4 oz. (114 gram) hummus (200 calories & 17 g carbs)

Day 11
- *Breakfast:* 1 serving Chia Seed Pudding (201 calories & 23 g carbs)
- *Snack:* 4 oz. (114 gram) apple + 1 tsp. nut butter (155 calories & 20 g carbs)

Day 12
- *Breakfast:* 1 serving Chia Seed Pudding + 2 eggs (345 calories & 24 g carbs)

- *Snack:* 5.2 oz (148 g) Greek yogurt (0%) + 1 oz. (29 g) almonds (248 calories & 12 g carbs)

Day 13
- *Breakfast:* 1 serving Protein Pancakes + 2 tsp. nut butter (372 calories & 24 g carbs)
- *Snack:* 1 serving Keto Peanut Butter Fat Bombs (247 calories & 3 g carbs)

Day 14
- *Breakfast:* 1 serving Cottage Cheese Pancakes + 1 tsp. nut butter (300 calories & 23 g carbs)
- *Snack:* 5 oz. (143 gram) Shelled edamame (200 calories & 14 g carbs)

Monthly Meal Plan

This is my personal monthly plan.

Week 1

- Day 1-2: Egg Muffins (352 calories & 8g carbs)
- Day 3: Cauliflower Oatmeal + 2 eggs (353 calories & 25g carbs)
- Day 4: Chia Seed Pudding (201 calories & 23g carbs)
- Day 5: Chia Seed Pudding + 2 eggs (345 calories & 24g carbs)

- Day 6: Protein Pancakes + 2 tsp nut butter (372 calories & 24g carbs)
- Day 7: Cottage Cheese Pancakes + 1 tsp nut butter (300 calories & 23g carbs)

Week 2

- Day 8-9: Egg Muffins (352 calories & 8g carbs)
- Day 10: Cauliflower Oatmeal + 2 eggs (353 calories & 25g carbs)
- Day 11: Chia Seed Pudding (201 calories & 23g carbs)
- Day 12: Chia Seed Pudding + 2 eggs (345 calories & 24g carbs)
- Day 13: Protein Pancakes + 2 tsp nut butter (372 calories & 24g carbs)
- Day 14: Cottage Cheese Pancakes + 1 tsp nut butter (300 calories & 23g carbs)

Week 3
- Day 15: Spinach Omelette (250 calories & 6g carbs)
- Day 16: Greek Yogurt Parfait (200 calories & 15g carbs)
- Day 17: Avocado Toast (320 calories & 10g carbs)
- Day 18: Smoothie Bowl (350 calories & 20g carbs)
- Day 19: Breakfast Burrito (300 calories & 15g carbs)
- Day 20: Cinnamon Rolls (250 calories & 20g carbs)

Week 4

- Day 21: Egg Muffins (352 calories & 8g carbs)
- Day 22: Cauliflower Oatmeal + 2 eggs (353 calories & 25g carbs)
- Day 23: Chia Seed Pudding (201 calories & 23g carbs)
- Day 24: Chia Seed Pudding + 2 eggs (345 calories & 24g carbs)
- Day 25: Protein Pancakes + 2 tsp nut butter (372 calories & 24g carbs)
- Day 26: Cottage Cheese Pancakes + 1 tsp nut butter (300 calories & 23g carbs)
- Day 27: Breakfast Tacos (250 calories & 10g carbs)
- Day 28: Omelette (200 calories & 6g carbs)
- Day 29: Breakfast Sandwich (300 calories & 15g carbs)
- Day 30: Waffles (250 calories & 20g carbs)

Note: The calorie and carb counts are approximate and may vary based on specific ingredients and portion sizes.

CONCLUSION

"Congratulations on taking the first step towards managing your diabetes and improving your overall health! This cookbook has provided you with 30 delicious and nutritious breakfast recipes specifically designed for individuals with diabetes.

Remember, breakfast is the most important meal of the day, and with these recipes, you can start your day off right. From egg muffins to chia seed pudding, and from protein pancakes to cottage cheese pancakes, we've got you covered.

Don't let diabetes hold you back from enjoying a tasty and satisfying breakfast. With the recipes in this cookbook, you can indulge in your favorite breakfast foods while still managing your blood sugar levels.

Remember to always consult with your healthcare provider or registered dietitian for personalized dietary advice, and don't hesitate to experiment with new ingredients and recipes to find what works best for you.

Happy cooking and happy eating! With the right tools and knowledge, you can take control of your diabetes and live a healthy and fulfilling life."

APPENDIX

USEFUL RESOURCES FOR MANAGING DIABETES

- *Diabetes ABCs*:

This refers to managing your blood glucose, blood pressure, and cholesterol levels. It may lower your chances of having health problems from diabetes, such as a heart attack, stroke, kidney disease, blindness and foot or leg amputations.

- *Healthy Meal Plan*:

 Work with your healthcare team to create a meal plan that works for you. You may need to eat smaller portions or enjoy your favorite foods less often.

- *Physical Activity*:

Physical activity may help you lower blood glucose, blood pressure and cholesterol levels. Being active may also help you get better sleep and improve your mood.

- *Medicine*:

Taking diabetes medicines is often part of managing diabetes. The medicines you take depend on your type of diabetes, how well medicines control your blood glucose level and other health conditions you may have.

- *Blood Glucose Meter*:

You can check your blood glucose level at home with a blood glucose meter. The meter tests a drop of your blood, usually from a prick of your fingertip. The meter will show you how much glucose is in your blood at that moment.

- *Diabetes Prevention Programs*:

Find out more about CDC-recognized Diabetes Prevention Programs in your area.

- *YMCA*:

Find out more about Diabetes Prevention Program support groups that may be in your area.

- *Diabetes Care Plan*:

Work with your healthcare team to create a diabetes care plan that works for you.

- *Health Checkups Tracker*:

Download the Health Checkups Tracker, which includes information you may want to track. You can take this information with you when you visit your healthcare team.

DIABETES ASSOCIATIONS AND ORGANIZATIONS

- *American Diabetes Association*:

Advocates and educates on all aspects of diabetes. Throughout the year, the ADA holds hundreds of events across the United States.

- *Juvenile Diabetes Research Foundation*:

The leading global organization funding innovative research to cure, prevent, and treat type 1 diabetes and its complications.

- *The Betes Organization*:

Developed to help people with diabetes address the mental and emotional health components of their condition using theater and puppetry.

- *We Are Diabetes*:

Offers a unique type of support—a one-on-one mentorship and resources to anyone with type 1 diabetes who also has an eating disorder.

- *Diabetes Research Institute Foundation*:

Created to cure diabetes. The mission and vision of the organization is to develop a biological cure by restoring natural insulin production and normalizing blood sugar levels without imposing other risks.
- *World Diabetes Foundation*: A global funder of diabetes prevention and care.

- *International Diabetes Federation*:

An umbrella organization of over 240 national diabetes associations in 160 countries and territories.

Recommended Books and Websites

Books:

- "The Easy Diabetes Cookbook" by Pam j.Rios
- "Mediterranean Dish Diet cookbook for Beginners 2024
-"Dash diet cookbook for Beginners 2024
 -" Diabetes Breakfast Recipes cookbook 2024
-"Renal Diet
-"Anti inflammatory diet
-"Heathy heart recipes
-"Vegan diet
All written by me, Read them.

Websites:

- American Diabetes Association (ADA)
- Juvenile Diabetes Research Foundation (JDRF)
- The Betes Organization
- We Are Diabetes
- Diabetes Research Institute Foundation
- World Diabetes Foundation
- International Diabetes Federation

These resources offer a range of recipes, meal plans, and cooking tips for managing diabetes, as well as information on nutrition, exercise, and lifestyle changes. They are written by registered dietitians, chefs, and healthcare professionals, and are suitable for individuals with diabetes, prediabetes, and gestational diabetes, as well as their families and caregivers.

Tracking Tools and Apps

1. *Glucose Tracking Apps*:
   - MySugr
   - Glucose Buddy
   - OneDrop
   - Glucosio
2. *Food Diary Apps:*
   - MyFitnessPal
   - Lose It!
   - Calorie Counter
   - Fooducate
3. *Blood Pressure and Weight Tracking Apps:*
   - MyNetDiary
   - Blood Pressure Companion
   - Weight Loss Tracker
4. *Exercise and Activity Tracking Apps:*
   - Fitbit
   - Apple Health
   - Google Fit
   - Strava
5. *Medication Reminders and Tracking Apps:*
   - Medisafe
   - MyMedSchedule

   - PillReminder
6. ***Carb Counting and Nutrition Apps:***
   - Carb Counter
   - Nutrition Facts
   - Calorie King
7. ***Diabetes Management Apps***:
   - OneTouch Reveal
   - Accu-Chek Connect
   - Dexcom CLARITY
8. ***Health and Wellness Apps:***
   - Headspace (meditation and mindfulness)
   - Sleep Cycle (sleep tracking)
   - Waterlogged (water intake tracking)

These tracking tools and apps can help you monitor and manage your condition, making it easier to stick to a healthy breakfast routine and overall lifestyle.

GLOSSARY

A1C (HbA1C) - A test that measures average blood glucose levels over the past 2-3 months.

Blood Glucose - The amount of glucose in the blood at a given time.

Carbohydrate - A type of macronutrient that raises blood glucose levels.

Carb Counting - A method of tracking carbohydrate intake to manage blood glucose levels.

Diabetes - A condition in which the body either cannot produce or effectively use insulin, a hormone that regulates blood glucose levels.

Exchange List - A system of grouping foods by carbohydrate, protein, and fat content to help with meal planning.

Fasting Blood Glucose - A test that measures blood glucose levels after an overnight fast.

Glucose - A simple sugar that serves as a primary source of energy for the body.

Glycemic Index (GI) - A ranking of carbohydrates based on how quickly they raise blood glucose levels.

Insulin - A hormone produced by the pancreas that regulates blood glucose levels.

Ketones - Substances produced when the body breaks down fat for energy instead of glucose.

Macronutrients - Carbohydrates, protein, and fat, which provide energy and support growth and maintenance of the body.

Net Carbs - The total carbohydrate content of a food minus the fiber and sugar alcohols.

Portion Control - Eating a specific amount of food to manage carbohydrate and calorie intake.

Prediabetes - A condition in which blood glucose levels are higher than normal but not high enough to be classified as diabetes.

Protein - A macronutrient that helps build and repair body tissues.

Sugar Alcohols - Low-calorie sweeteners that do not raise blood glucose levels.

Type 1 Diabetes - An autoimmune disease in which the body does not produce insulin.

Type 2 Diabetes - A condition in which the body does not effectively use insulin.

This glossary provides definitions for key terms related to diabetes, nutrition, and meal planning, helping you understand the concepts and terminology used in the book.

ABOUT THE AUTHOR

PAM J. RIOS is a registered dietician and diabetes educator with over 20 years of experience helping people manage their diabetes through diet and lifestyle changes. She has a personal connection to diabetes, having been diagnosed with type 2 diabetes herself in her 40s. After struggling to manage her condition through conventional treatments, Pam discovered the Mediterranean diet and found that it was the key to reversing her diabetes and regaining her health. She is now passionate about sharing her knowledge and experience with others through her writing and work as a diabetes educator. Pam is also the author of several other books on diabetes and nutrition. Check them out. Dash diet cookbook for Beginners 2024, Mediterranean Dish Diet cookbook for Beginners 2024 and many others.its definitely a must read for all.

I Care alot..